The Toybag Guide to

Age Play

by Lee "Bridgett" Harrington

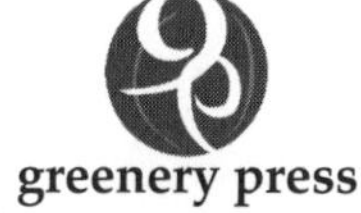

Published in the United States by Greenery Press, 4200 Park Blvd. pmb 240, Oakland, CA 94602, www.greenerypress.com.

ISBN 1-890159-73-5.

CONTENTS

Readers should understand that all BDSM carries an inherent risk of physical injury, emotional injury, injury to relationships, and other types of harm. While we believe that following the guidelines set forth in this book will help you reduce that risk to a reasonable level, the writer and publisher encourage you to understand that you are choosing to take some risk when you decide to engage in these activities, and to accept personal responsibility for that risk.

While we have diligently researched the information we put in this book, it may nonetheless be incomplete, inaccurate, or out of date. Therefore, in acting on the information in this book, you agree to accept its contents "as is" and "with all faults." Please notify us of any errors so that we may address them in future printings.

The information in this book should not be used as medical or therapeutic advice. Neither the author, the publisher nor anyone else associated with the creation or sale of this book is liable for any damage caused by your participating in the activities described herein.

Introduction: Or, What Brought Me to Age Play.

When I was pretty young I started taking care of the people around me, or being a big mean bully — it really depended on the group of kids I was around, and what sort of power dynamic I wanted to establish. But either way I was always the biggest, always the one who knew what was going on, the one who found the neatest cheap or free toys and then passed them out around the neighborhood. I grew up in a challenging neighborhood, with gang fights and turf issues, while going to school in a highly affluent neighborhood because that's where "kids like me had a right to go." Class issues, just another power dynamic, came to me at an early age as a lower-middle-class kid with a high IQ score.

As the years went by, I started to obsess about taking care of the folks around me. When I was a street teen punk (back in the bad years), I was the kid who always sobered up in a snap when the cops came around, made sure everyone made it somewhere safe to crash for the night, even if it meant taking the last five dollars out of my pocket. It came as a surprise to no one that I became a summer camp counselor, but it didn't last long because by the end of the summer I'd had a fling with a girl at camp — an issue because though she was older than me, she was a camper and I was not, so I was out.

When I first started exploring BDSM (Bondage/Discipline; Dominance/Submission; Sadism/Masochism), as a teenager, it was laid out for me very clearly by someone who believed in the "one true way" that as a young person in the scene I could only be a bottom. I only had the right to bottom until I had learned everything, then I would be given my first leather, my first flogger, my first bottom to practice on. I look back on those years and those traditions and am grateful for them, but I also wonder if being told that only older people could be as lovingly cruel as I longed to be was the capper on my nascent age play fetish.

After a few years of exploring with partners outside of the public eye of clubs, social gatherings, and kinky conferences, I finally joined the "dark world of perversion," known as "the scene," in 1995. It was a bit of a letdown at first. Here I'd built up this huge mystique around the taboo of playing these power games in a pubic arena, dreaming of dark dungeons and miles of leathermen in tight chaps and women whose heels made them a thousand feet tall. I was pleasantly surprised that once I got over the fact that a lot of the attendees in Seattle just showed up wearing denim jeans and black teeshirts (but oh such immaculate leather boots), I actually learned something.

I learned that the one true way I had been taught was not the only way.

I learned that slaves, boys, servants, grrrls, and bottoms had the right to say No! I learned that there were a thousand forms of fantasy being enacted by thousands of imaginative souls. And... I learned I wasn't the only one who wanted to enact the power games that age roleplay offered me.

I made my first public forays into age roleplay, which is more commonly referred to as "age play," in one of the most acceptable forms possible for a teenager blessed with a huge rack — the schoolgirl. I wriggled into a plaid skirt, a tight button-down white shirt over a white lace bra, white panties, knee high white socks, a pair of Converse high top sneakers, pinned my hair out of my face with bows, and was ready to blow a few minds. OK, I wasn't planning on blowing any minds, just trying to impress a few folks with how gosh-darn cute I was.

It worked. The mystique of the adult dressed like a schoolgirl had folks of all genders and orientations stepping into roles unconsciously. Some became teachers and principals, asking if I'd been a good girl or if I needed a spanking. Some became bratty boys and girls and picked on me or let me untie their shoes. Some whispered secrets in my ears. And a few dirty old men (and one dirty hot woman who ran Beyond the Edge Café, where we were meeting at the time) asked if I needed some candy.

My internal dialogue (aka what I jerked off in bed to) of what was hot about age dynamics was not being a teenage strumpet in plaid. But it worked. And it opened the door for me that yes, this could be OK. Not only was it OK, but other people were doing it already, consciously and unconsciously.

The private exploration started with the Leather Master/boy dynamic, and the public one began with the Teacher/schoolgirl one. From there I became a Boy Scout, the neighborhood bully, the erotic initiator of a fellow youth, the sexy step-sister, the altar boy. But I was stuck in the perception that because I was still young, I had to follow in the mold of the "one true way" I'd first been shown. And then, one night in bed with a lover, it happened. He was being sweet and getting us water after a hot bout of all night sweaty sex, and came back into the room eating a cookie.

"Did I say you could have a cookie, young man?"

"Um, no.... Ma'am?"

"Do I need to teach you a lesson?"

"No, I mean, I won't do it again, I mean..." and he stammered over his own words trying to figure out what the hell he'd just walked into.

The scene progressed as I, the evil manipulative babysitter, requiring the "young boy" to do sexual favors for me unless I told on him for eating cookies after bedtime. The young man was nearly forty.

From there I learned I could play all over the board. I played with the Principal's office and the Boot training camp for young impressionable men. I enjoyed a wide variety of activities and roles, including getting to be Santa in bed for a certain naughty young lady.

But I never understood a few types of age play I saw mentioned when looking for online porn or talking with others who enjoyed these sorts of games: Daddy/Mommy play and Infantilism.

Oh, I understood why each could be hot! But knowing the rules of Rugby does not give you much of an insight into why during the World Cup people take days at a time off of work to stay up and watch matches in different time zones, while painted absurd colors and screaming at the top of their lungs. I had a few fantasies about each of those concepts, but had convinced myself that "Only needy men with issues about power wear diapers" or "All people who enact Daddy scenes were obviously abused as children." Neither is the case.

Yes, there are some individuals who fall into those categories, as we will address later in this book, but they are far from the majority on any sort of age play. In 2006, after 14 years of exploring age play dynamics with lovers, both concepts finally clicked.

I had insisted for years that I would never be a Daddy or Mommy, and that I would always be Aunty, Uncle, Babysitter, Cousin… but never that. But then, in the shower after a long day and night of play (sound familiar?), my partner was in the shower and I climbed in behind him. I reached for the soap, and as water cascaded down his wide back, I heard the sweetest tones escape my lips.

"Here, honey, let me get your back for you."

And his voice went up, scared, unsure…

"Is this okay, Mummy?"

I melted, not because he said the words, but because he had picked up on the fact that I had gone there first. I shushed him, and said be quiet, we don't want the neighbors to hear. Thus began a torrid steamy scene that lasted about thirty minutes, involved a lot of sudsy soap as a lubricant, eager fingers and moans caught between words that left us both toasty — and confused.

What the hell had just happened? We sat and talked about whether this was enacting some weird abuse cycle from either of our pasts, and nope, this didn't hit any of our "bad" buttons. We tried to figure out where it came from. Then we shut up for a moment, kissed, and asked each other if we wanted to go for another round or roleplay. Yes, yes, we both did.

Age roleplay, or age play, is not for everyone, but it is also not a "precursor to pedophilia." In the following pages we will dive into such a wide variety of roles, activities, and sensibilities that I bet most of you will find at least one thing that appeals. Have you ever considered roleplaying that you are nineteen years old and sneaking into a club? What about individuals who enjoy pretending to be older? Fetishizing the age they are right now? We'll cover all of these, along with concepts of archetypes, power dynamics, types of interactions, and of course... how to make it yours.

So, slip on your favorite smoking jacket, button up your crisp white blouse, dig out your favorite stuffed teddy bear, or just pour yourself something to drink... and let's dive in together into the wide world of fantasy that is AGE PLAY.

Chapter One. What is Age Play?

I get asked all the time what Age Play is. It can mean a thousand things to a thousand different sexual adventurers or curious roleplaying enthusiasts, but there are key threads that run through it.

Age play is any interaction or roleplay between consenting adults (or enjoyed by a solo adult) involving the concept of age as a dynamic. Wow — that's a lot of stuff. This can include but is not limited to:

— age regression back to being a "kid" (pretending to be 7 and playing video games or masturbating for the first time)

— fetishizing one's current age (the power of being a twenty-year-old woman)

— age forwarding towards being a different age bracket (a thirty-year-old dressing up to be Santa Claus)

— or any roleplay interacting with any of these concepts.

Age play incorporates a sensual or sexual element, but many "age players," "kidz," "babiez," or "littles" enjoy "pure" age play that is just about the role and not about any hanky-panky.

Age play is not pedophilia, child porn, or individuals interested in playing with actual biological children. Age Players may use the props of "bio kids" but we are into the props and trappings, not the kids themselves in any way.

Why do age play?

Can you remember how much fun it was to forget about your homework and just run outside and play? How about how the butterflies in your stomach you felt the first time you had a crush on someone? What about remembering trying to learn something new and feeling so proud when your own parents said, "Way to go!"

It is for these feelings and more that many individuals are tantalized by age roleplay. We live in a world where day-to-day stress, from the office to the home environment, occupies our every waking moment. We live in a world without enough touch or joy. We have been so sucked into our banality that we forget the pure exuberance we experienced as children... and it's time we reclaimed that. There are a thousand ways to reclaim that joy (or, for some of us, to build joy where very little happened before in our lives), but age play can be an amazing tool not just for that, but for adding spice to one's sex life as well.

I've talked with a wide range of age players. Here are some, but far from all, of the reasons we have gotten into age play, either as "kidz" or as "adultz":

Having fun or being silly

Dressing up

Connecting with a partner in a different way

Building trust or being trusted

Letting go of stress

Reliving childhood

Taboo

Reclaiming/rewriting childhood

Spontaneity

Enjoying a physical activity (jump rope, spankings, sex)

Sense of innocence

"Corrupting" someone

Emotional exploration

Giving up/gaining control

Sensual/sexual foreplay

Doing things "you" wouldn't normally do

Enjoying a special event

Brattiness/feistiness

Enjoying a fetish object (heels, stockings, white socks)

Physical restraint or struggling

Being casual/ fun when hanging out with friends

Adding spice to a relationship

Providing service

Inner identity

Gender exploration

Dominance/submission

Relationship structure

Acting as a teacher/guardian

Getting a chance to grow up all over again

Never having to grow up

Might any of these call out to you? Not all of them have to. Just one is enough to consider exploring this exciting world of fantasy exploration.

Archetypes for Age Play

Later in this book we will explore a wide variety of archetypes or templates for how to actually do age play. However, the first thing we need to consider is what kind of archetype we are enacting.

An archetype is a template, a pattern, that we will never perfectly fit. Almost all roleplay, be it on the playground or in the bedroom, begins with an archetype. Doctor/patient roleplay when you were a child enacted an archetype of what your culture considered to be "traditional" behavior for those roles, and then you made them your own. However, with age play there are three major forms of archetypes that we can explore, and each has their own merits and pitfalls to take into consideration.

UNIVERSAL ARCHETYPES

In every culture around the world, universal archetypes exist. These are the templates of our collective unconscious, and are the perfect ideals that exist in the back of our brains. Examples of universal archetypes include Father, Mother, Hunter, Child, Hermit, Righteous Ruler, Cruel Ruler… they are the human experiences that have repeated themselves over and over again in our mammalian brain.

If we are choosing to take on the universal archetype of "Mother," she is the nurturer from which we all came,

Gaia, Mother Earth, the perfect nurturer and caregiver, the womb of the universe. She has been transformed through cultural lenses into a thousand shapes: Isis, Demeter, Mary. The universal archetype of "Father," on the other hand, is all-knowing, strong, independent, an educator, he who leads by example. In cultural views the universal archetype of Father has been seen as Osiris, Zeus, Yahweh.

Cultural archetypes

Technically, each of the facets of a universal archetype as seen through our cultural experience is a cultural archetype, but that definition is far too broad for our exploration of age play. What I mean by Cultural Archetype exploration in age roleplay is the idea of common experiences of age dynamics in our media and culture that we grew up with, or live with now.

For example, for individuals growing up in the United States during the 1950s, June and Ward Cleaver are archetypal parents, with Beaver being an archetypal media child. If we fast-forward to the 1980s, we replace the experience of the mother in the polka dots with the Cosby family, where Mrs. Cosby was no-nonsense, had a full -time job, and was going to keep her kids in line even if it meant hard love and depriving them of pudding.

Television is just one example of where we can find cultural archetypes. Books provide us with an amazing array of archetypes to choose from — Alice Through the Looking Glass, the powerful mix of children, heroes and villains presented in the Harry Potter novels or C.S. Lewis' work, and how can we forget classics like wild child Huckleberry Finn? Movies show us examples of powerful adults and children alike — from the quirky Willy Wonka to the terrifying monster adults in movies such as Saw and Texas Chainsaw Massacre.

And let's not forget our newspapers and nightly news! Pop culture icons, young and old, provide us with a bevy of roles to consider exploring: Santa Claus, Paris Hilton, The Royal Families, Celebrities, MILFs (Mothers I'd Like to Fuck) and Cougars (older women who go looking for younger men) on Oprah. All of these and more can give us a great springboard for our fantasy life.

Personal archetypes

Unlike cultural or universal archetypes, personal archetypes cannot be viewed in books or magazines. They are the caricatures of the people we actually have known or who have been part of our life in some other way. We long to be as bratty as our cousin Sally used to be when we got together after school. We draw upon the memory of our high school math teacher to inspire a strict yet loving teacher archetype. We giggle at the opportunity to have our lover role-play the persona of the person who was our first kiss.

Personal archetypes are at the same time both the most common type of archetype used in roleplay, but they are also the most challenging to navigate. If everyone involved in a roleplay experience has read a novel, we all know what happened before and after in the story surrounding the point that we want to experience in the moment. But in personal tales we are drawing from, there is a danger of emotional land mines. If we ask our partner to roleplay back to the time when we were just thirteen years old and about to have our first kiss, our partner may not know that after the first kiss that same person left us heartbroken, and that in reliving that experience we are somehow hoping they can fix the memory. If we don't share that knowledge with our partner, we're asking them to be psychic, which is unfair to them and to us.

My favorite use for personal archetypes is to use them as inspiration, not to replicate exact memories. I love pulling on the memories of my favorite drama teacher to be a quirky gay man, who in my fantasy life seduces the senior high school student director. I enjoy remembering my first camp crush, Barbara, and using her as a template for taking on her adventurous spirit and ability to conquer all obstacles. I can challenge myself to become a caricature of my creepy uncle, my strong-as-steel mother, or the scary cop who arrested me for attempted shoplifting when I was a teen.

Notice that I am challenging myself to take on these roles, not asking my partner to take them on? Unless our partner was there and has met the people of our own life drama, how can they capture the essence of the archetypes from my life? Yes, they can pull from the stories that we have told, but understand that they will take your stories and make them their own, pulling upon the archetypes from their own life to fill in the gaps.

When archetypes collide

Personal archetypes can also be a dangerous area to play in for anyone who has ever had childhood traumas... and to be honest, there are few of us who have not had some sort of life trauma. When a lover starts asking me to call them specific pet names that we have not used before, while doing a specific sexual activity, warning bells start going off for me. Some individuals use age roleplay as an opportunity to re-open old wounds, consciously or unconsciously. I find that though therapeutic, roleplay is not therapy. We will address this issue later in this text, but be aware of not just your partners' behaviors, but your own. Are you pulling upon personal archetypes to relive a fun memory, or to create something enjoyable from the caricatures of your life, or are you trying to have them replicate behaviors from past traumas?

If the answer is that you are trying to relive, replicate or touch on past traumas, it does not mean you can not do that sort of roleplay. However, I would highly recommend discussing these issues openly with your partner in advance so that they are aware of what they are getting into, or choosing not to get into. However, not everyone knows they are going to open up old war wounds — your partner may use a specific string of words pulling from a cultural archetype of being the "Bad Uncle," not knowing that someone in your own life used that same series of statements to harm you in your own life. People can unknowingly play into our own personal archetypes, but be aware that most of the time, it is not purposefully done, and if we just step out of role for a moment the damage can be undone. (We'll discuss this more presently.)

Another common miscommunication happens when discussing what type of age play to do. Many folks experience breakdowns in communication about age play at this point because one person says I want you to be a Daddy for me (cultural archetype), and the partner says how can I be a Daddy?

— my father was a horrid man (personal archetype).

This is when the skill set of "active listening" comes in handy. The first partner asked for the second partner to be "a Daddy." They did not ask for them to be "just like my father," or "just like your father." It can seem daunting to try to figure out what your partner means when such loaded terms come into play, but I find that the terms that make us squirm the most or challenge our abilities often have the most rewards waiting after the struggle is done.

Chapter Two. So you've decided to give it a try...

Having read this far into the book, or having fantasized for years about pretending to be a naughty schoolgirl or dirty old man, you've decided it's time to give it a try. Maybe you've been doing this for years already, and this book is just giving you new ways to examine your current play. Fabulous! The question is, where do we go from here?

Levels of investment

The first question I usually ask people interested in playing with me involving some sort of age roleplay dynamic, is: "How much investment do you want to put into this?" They often look at me baffled, so let me explain with a few basic levels. There are, of course, levels between these, but consider this the start of discussing your desires:

— Three-Minute Roleplay. This is the level where you are fooling around in bed, and someone says playfully "ooooh, headmistress, may I have a spanking?" The partner looks back, giggles, throws the partner over her lap, and after five slaps, the roleplay is over. There is no emotional investment in the role, just one or more people trying on a role for the fun of it, then going on with life.

— Scene/Evening Investment. Taking the above example, the two partners had fun with the role, and decide that on Friday night, they are going to play more fully with it. After getting home from work, both of them have dinner together, then each goes into the bedroom and gets changed. He wriggles into short pants he found at a garage sale and a shirt that he used to wear at work, while she throws on a really severe skirt from the last funeral she went to and a pink button-down blouse that was buried in the closet. They begin verbal banter, which turns into the "boy" having to write his apologies 200 times in a notebook, then receives his spankings while saying “thank you, headmistress,” before the headmistress says he can make it up to her by showing him a good time after school. The two of them turn back into just being lovers somewhere around the second or third orgasm, and both cuddle up to sleep having had a fun time that may never be done again: it was just something to spice up their sex life.

A scene/evening investment is just that — no serious money spent, no long hours coming up with perfect persona names, and if it all goes horribly, you can go back to doing what you already do well together. The only investment is time, whether it be three hours at a club, an evening at home, or heading out together to the zoo to be ten-year-olds together while looking at zebras.

— Repeat Role. This level of investment happens after the same scene or characters have been done more than once. Patterns of interaction are established, such as the school boy knowing that every time Mistress asks a question, he needs to reply with short answers such as "Yes Headmistress" or "No Headmistress." Perhaps the role that has been done over and over is two "teenage boys" (in reality thirty-year-old men) jerking each other off in a semi public place, and if so perhaps the pattern of interaction established is that both partners know that the roleplay has begun as soon as a specific wink or smirk has happened. At this level of investment, props also start to take on a power of their own. As soon as the woman in the first interaction slides into that pink blouse she usually hates, suddenly she feels a bit more like the sensual and cruel Headmistress. As soon as the "teens" get into their faded and torn jeans, they remember the heat of what it was like to have taboo sexuality back in their small towns.

— Personal Investment. I like to call this category "when your hobby starts spending your money." I cannot count the sheer quantity of props I have accumulated over the years because of personae I became attached to. Lacy underwear that matched a cooking apron for being a Mommy. The perfect tie for my Daddy. A perfectly curved rattan cane to gift the delicious Nanny who used to play with me.

When we're at this level of investment, we have started to think about the role when not in role. We wander down the street and think, ooh, that object would be great for our play. We contemplate what we would like to do next when in persona. We start signing our emails in our persona name rather than our actual name. And since we're not just thinking about the role when in role, it starts to get imbued with a certain degree of intimacy as well. It becomes part of us, and if our partner decides that they no longer want to play with "Santa," we are hurt because we feel like we were rejected, even if it was just the persona that no longer holds an attraction for our partners.

— Full-Time Identity. In this final degree of investment, individuals transform their roles into the full-time basis for their relationships. Daddy/boy relationships become full-time mentoring and supporting relationships, even if the boy still holds a job. Mommy/girl relationships often take on a caretaking and nurturing structure, and use the terms Mommy and girl outside of the bedroom. Sister relationships that may have started as two women being there to brush each other's hair have now become full-time family for one another, with all its ups and downs, even if there is no biological tie. Also known as a 24/7 relationship, full-time identity investment takes a lot of negation and communication skills for all individuals involved to make sure that the "kidz" get their needs met, since they are still adults at the end of the day.

There is no "better" level of investment. There is no reason for individuals to strive towards full-time roleplay dynamics when they and their partners are happy to repeat roles. Take a moment, breathe, have fun, and be in the moment. See what you can gain from what makes both you and your partner happy instead of pushing for something else just because it seems more intense. Sometimes the most magical moments come when we aren't looking for them.

"Ages" of Kidz

Each age category has its own merits, and different individuals prefer playing in different categories of age.

I enjoy playing with a variety of categories depending on who my partner is, how hard my day at work was, and how nicely my lover asks.

— Pre-Verbal. Also known as Infantilism, this category of play involves an adult, usually in diapers or nude, with an "adult" they trust. Pre-verbal individuals have to trust implicitly that they are in good hands, because if they are roleplaying that they can't speak, how can they say "no"? Common themes and activities include humiliation, "babying," spoiling, bottle feeding, breast worship, innocence, and the power inherent in becoming a very young child for a period of time.

— Toddler. From the "terrible twos" up until they enter school, adults who want to be this age often enjoy physical activity, learning new things, potty training, candy, and exploring gender stereotypes. This is the persona age when we start learning about innies and outies, sharing our toys, family dynamics, messy food play, and bed time stories.

— School Kid. This is a wide age category, and starts as we "enter school" up until we hit puberty. School Kid personas learn about team sports, school subjects, scouting, summer camp, doctors, "cooties," and best friends.

— Teen. The most common age play theme is fueled by the fact that this time period in most lives was so fraught with sexual tension. From rebels to teacher's pets, Lolita seduction artists to bullies and first clumsy kisses, this age category is rife with opportunities for exploration, from innocent to sadistic.

— Post-teen/Adult. It may not seem like a "kid" category, but the reality is that age power dynamics do exist beyond the teen years. Examples include pretending to be twenty years old sneaking into a bar in Los Angeles, the "adult" Boy in service to "Grandma," and a variety of college/university themes.

Roles for "Adultz"

Why should kidz have all the fun in choosing personas? There are a wide variety of roles and personas or adultz to choose from as well!

— Mommy/Momma/Mom or Daddy/Poppa/Dad. One of the most common of age play adult terms is also the most challenging for many people to parse. For many of us, the idea of using a term associated with our own parental figures leads us to question whether we have some sort of Oedipus complex, and that can be distracting or even disturbing. For others, if there was any sort of history of childhood trauma associated with a specific parent, using a term associated with that parent can not only be challenging, but harmful for the psyche. For that reason I strongly recommend, unless you are very sure of yourself, that you consider using a term that was not part of your own or your "kidz" childhood experience. Perhaps Father and Dad are loaded terms, but is Poppa, Papa, Padre or Daddy? This type of Adult role can often lead to a need to caretake or look after your "kid," so be forewarned that for many individuals who use these terms, emotional bonds may form faster than expected.

— Extended Adult Family. From Aunties and Uncles to Cousins, Grandparents, Step-Parents and Third Cousins Twice Removed, there is a wide variety of personae to choose from. If familial play (aka incest roleplay) really appeals for taboo reasons, but Mommy and Daddy make people uncomfortable, playing around with personas like the quirky Aunt or the lewd Granny can work for many people as a way to have fun — especially if they don't have any biological counterparts!

— Daily Roles. This category of Adultz were the people we see daily or on a very regular basis. They can include the babysitter, teacher, coach, next-door neighbor, or bus driver. Regular roles in our lives offer a variety of roleplaying situations (teacher can spoil us, can punish us, can invite us home for private lessons) without invoking the taboo of incest. For many people, the taboo of age roleplay is hard enough to play with. These sorts of role also take away the idea that this role will last "forever." Teachers get transferred, and babysitters quit. We might miss them, but things can end. We can get a new teacher, even if the new teacher will never be the same — but if Daddy leaves us, it can be heartbreaking.

— Special Time Roles. This category of Adultz were the people we only saw on an irregular basis, and thus time with them can be all the more special or terrifying. Examples include the doctor, dentist, camp counselor, priest, and ice cream vendor. These are great roles for play partners we only get to see once a year, or with whom we have never explored this sort of role. They can also be a fun second role for individuals who want to continue doing age roleplay, but need a break from their regular role.

— The Stranger. Perhaps the scariest and yet often very tantalizing category for many individuals, especially those from the BDSM community who want to start exploring age play, is the idea of strangers interacting with kidz. From the kidnapper to rapist, seductress (hello Mrs. Robinson) to drug dealer, strangers can offer a wide variety of roles for fear and terror play. Strangers don't have to be all bad, though — what about the nice old lady who you can help across the street, or the man from France the teenage girl meets on a flight to visit her grandparents? There are as many possibilities as you can dream up — but remember, when playing with terrifying persona templates, the possibilities for emotional landmines do exist.

Interactions between Adultz and Kidz

When most individuals consider starting out with age roleplay, the first interaction dynamic that usually springs to mind that of the single adult (parent, teacher, priest) and a single kid. But why let our creativity end there, when so many other possibilities exist?

— Solo Kid. Yup, that's right. No adult has to be around for you to spend some quality time being a kid. Wake up, keep your pajamas on, and go watch Saturday morning cartoons! Go take a nap. Play your favorite computer game. Buy yourself that Barbie doll you always dreamed of owning. Go ahead, you deserve a date with yourself.

— Single Adult, Single Kid. From bedtime stories with Mommy to learning to fly a kite with Daddy, coloring with the babysitter or having a philosophical argument with your favorite teacher, the possibilities are endless.

— Single Adult, Family Tie Kidz. One of my favorite times is me and my "step-sister" getting to curl up on the couch, one on each side, and watch movies with Daddy. Other options include one ".parent" taking care of all the cousins, or another great, single-parent family dinner.

— Single Adult, Assorted Kidz. From scout gatherings to daycare, role play opportunities are common ageplay fantasies. Teacher with a class of students, Principal's office punishments, and the sports coach with the entire team are also good fun.

— Multiple Adultz, Single Kid. Time with Mommy and Daddy together is a great way for a couple to bring someone new (the kid) into their roleplaying. Perhaps you know someone with a medical fetish? If so, what about arranging for little Bobby to get to visit the nice nurses and doctors who will all poke and prod him?

— Multiple Adultz, Multiple Kidz. Okay, I admit, once this many people get involved, it can be a logistical nightmare — but worth it! From summer camp to zoo outings, family outings to company barbeques, community gatherings of age players can be an absolute joy.

— Kidz and Petz. In this case I am referring to human animal roleplaying — instead of pretending to be older or younger, or fetishizing their current age, some individuals enjoy roleplaying that they are a puppy, cat, horse, or other creature. What little boy hasn't always wanted a dog, and little girl longed to own a pony? Isn't it even better when that puppy or pony is your partner? So much easier to clean up after!

- Pair of Kidz. I can think of a few great ones that I've done: back seat fumbling, doing homework together, sibling rivalry, bully and the nerd, Princess and her lackey... what can you think of?

- Group of Kidz. Again, the co-ordination takes a fair amount of work, but when planning for these sorts of outings comes together, it is absolutely amazing. I've heard of scenes involving gangs, rites of passages, school dorm roleplay, popular kids with the nerd, and girls club with a solo boy trying to sneak in, and more.

— Multi Generation. Every Daddy needs a Daddy of his own. I have seen some truly amazing age play families form over the years, with rituals and hierarchies that work for them. Grandma, Dad and Kid all go shopping, or perhaps quirky Grandpa comes for a visit.

Chapter Three. Types of Scene

Every roleplay scenario that takes place can be called a "scene." This terminology can be confusing for some people because "the scene," collectively, can also be a term used for all individuals who publicly engage in BDSM and fantasy exchange. However, for our discussion, we will be using the first definition. So — how sexual and sensual should age play scenes be? This is a never-ending debate within the age play community, and my only answer is that each person who engages in age roleplay needs to make a decision for themselves. This needs to be discussed before roleplay begins, however, because it can be very damaging for a relationship if the first person believed the roleplay would be completely non-sexual while the other person believed it was supposed to be a "forced sexuality" roleplay scenario.

— Non-Sexual. Examples of non-sexual scenes include just about anything a bio-kid might do with the adults in their lives, from playing with blocks to going shopping, eating breakfast to doing homework. All of these activities can become sexualized or sensualized scenes. The point of non-sexual scenes is to simply enjoy the activities taking place, not to add sexual tension to the experience.

— Body Care and Grooming. These sorts of scenes, including bathing, dressing and brushing hair, often have a sensual overtone. Light touches become loving caresses as we clip in bows, wash hair, and praise our little ones on how charming they look.

— Solo Sexual. Tucking in my "little boy" after bedtime stories is not necessarily a sexual scene, but if after I leave, he chooses to continue the roleplay while alone in bed by masturbating, it becomes a solo sexual scene. Solo sexual scenes can also be seen as one-sided sexual tension, such as the school teacher walking in on the "baby dyke" reading the pornographic magazine, or the priest spying on the "young men" in his care.

— Consensual Sexual. My favorite consensual sexual scene is a pair of kidz fooling around with each other for their first time. Many of us remember the magic of our early sexual explorations, and it's a great way to recall those memories or build new ones. Other consensual sexual age play scenes include "incest" roleplay scenes that begin organically with little coercion, or experienced teenager relationships fooling around at the school dance.

— "Coerced" Sexual. Adult power over the lives of children might be seen by their nature to always be seen as coerced sexuality, but these scenes capitalize on the sexual tension involved in that coercion and don't just incorporate it, but thrive on that power dynamic. It doesn't have to be the Adult doing the coercion either. Lolita is an amazing archetype of the younger role taking the reins in roleplay. Or what about a group of teenage boys convincing the least popular boy to do something he doesn't want to? It is crucial to note that in any sort of "coerced" sexual scene, all players are in fact consenting adults who want to engage in the fantasy of coercion, and are not in fact being coerced into sexual activities.

— "Forced" Sexual. For many people, this is the most offensive concept of all in age play, but many individuals I have met over the years enjoy the fantasy of having their power taken from them in sexual situations, even if in reality they gave it up willingly and are in fact consenting ahead of time to all of the activities they are partaking in. Examples of forced sexual scenes are rape play (an offensive term to many, but it refers to individuals enacting roleplay of forced sex, and no actual rape is involved), extortion (if you suck my cock I won't have to tell your Daddy), and "underage prostitution." In any of these scenes, all players are in fact consenting adults who want to engage in the fantasy of forced sexuality, and are not in fact being forced into sexual activities.

— BDSM or Bondage. Some visuals come easily — the woman in a school girl uniform being bent over a desk and given 10 hard cane strokes by her husband dressed as the English schoolmaster, for example. Others require some creativity — Cowboys and Indians? Playground Bully? Drunk Daddy? Where does your fantasy life take you?

As you can see, the range of roles you have to choose from, as well as levels of interaction and types of scenes, are wide. What jumps out at you as hot? Scary? Fun? Terrifying? What might you want to try?

Chapter Four. Notes from the Playground.

I've learned from the many years I've been engaged in age play that the pick-and-choose system from the previous chapter works, but it is not the be-all end-all of what you should know if you really want to explore what age play has to offer. So let me give you some of the insights I've learned over the past decade of this sort of fantasy exploration for other types of age play you might not have considered, or to how to keep it special, fun, and functional in your relationship.

Who says all kidz are bottoms?

Not me! The stereotype in media is that in all age play, the "adult" is the dominant individual and the "kid" is the submissive. There is a belief that everyone who wants to roleplay as a kid is a "bottom" and has a desire to be spanked, or receive some other sort of physical pain. I have found that though this is true for some age play kidz, it is not a blanket statement. Many kidz I know are dominant princesses, enjoy wielding the brush for spanking their "teacher," or have no interest in physical pain play whatsoever.

Gender and age play

Every full grown woman longs to be a little girl, and every man wants to become a little boy, right? Not so. Many individuals enjoy the opportunity to explore gender roleplay along with their age play, with men having an opportunity to be little girls, teenage prima donnas, or mommies, while I know many women who enjoy being babies in blue, boys on the playground, or daddies. A heterosexual couple I know enjoy having the opportunity to be lesbian kidz fooling around together. Numerous transsexual friends of mine have used age play as an opportunity to get to relive their childhood in their gender of personal truth. Age play can be an amazing tool to explore gender roles, personal identity, and work beyond the perceived limits of our biology.

Aging the other direction

Who says biological age determines roles? My first little boy was twenty years my senior. I know many young adults who enjoy the opportunity to take on caretaker or other adult roles in their roleplay or lifestyle choices, just as I know many individuals who have raised biological grandchildren, yet who enjoy being little from time to time. Just because one partner is biologically older that the other, it does not mean they have to be the Adult in your roleplay.

In addition, I have had an opportunity to spend time with a number of individuals who enjoy taking age roleplay in the opposite direction of the littlez the words age play usually evoke. Known as "gerries," "elder players," or geriatric fetishists, these individuals enjoy forwarding their age to where they can roleplay being at the other end of the age spectrum. For some it is about perceived helplessness, being in need of medical assistance or caretakers due to lack of mental wherewithal. For others it is about exploring the props of that age group, from wheelchairs and canes to catheters and soft foods. I myself have enjoyed this type of roleplay as an opportunity to pretend for an evening to be a dirty old man luring young men into my bed out of sympathy or coercion... but maybe I'm just a dirty old man ahead of my time.

What about diapers?

There are two major categories of age players who tend to use adult diapers as part of their erotic role play — adult babiez and gerries.

However, the psychology of these two uses of diapers in play is very different. Diapers when being an Adult Baby (also called AB for short, or Infantilism in more technical terms) is often about being cared for, being too young to understand, the helplessness that comes from dependence to an authority figure or caretaker, and more. For Elder players, this feeling of helplessness is often loaded with a different set of role-playing fodder — the idea of no longer being able to care for oneself, incontinence, and embarrassment.

Available in most medical supply shops and online as "incontinence Briefs," adult diapers are in fact built for just that, taking care of bodily functions for individuals who are unable to control their bladder. There are also specialty retailers who make cloth adult diapers for individuals who prefer a more natural feel.

Do all people who wear diapers like to do golden (piss) or brown (scat) play? Not at all. In fact, there are all kinds of reasons to enjoy diapers. They can be a fun dress-up item, a fetish object, or something you can ejaculate in without making a mess. Other people I know do "fake" messy diapers, pouring lemonade or pudding in their drawers before being "discovered."

If diaper play appeals to you or your partner, I recommend that both of you take some time to discuss it out of role if possible. Many people are initially a bit freaked out by the idea of diapers, and it's best to discuss your desires and expectations outside the heat of the moment.

THE MIX AND MATCH GAME

So you like latex, and your partner likes age play — why not mix and match your desires so that everyone has a good time? You dress up as the latex nurse, they can slip on a latex school girl outfit, and everyone has a great time! Consider playing Cowboys and Indians to satisfy bondage enthusiasts. A wide variety of fetishes, fantasies and desires mix very well with age play. Put your thinking cap on and look at how you could mix and match age play with pain play, sensations and sensuality, golden showers (piss play), enemas, lactation, sexuality of all stripes, dirty talking, domestic service, dominance and submission, medical fetish, tickling, wet and messy food... and so much more.

Chapter Five. Being a Unique Little Snowflake.

Everyone deserves to feel special. Coming up with pet names and age roleplay terms that refer to your relationship and your relationship alone are an amazing tool for making that roleplay dynamic as unique as it truly is. Perhaps finding toys that are only used with one partner (paddles, Daddy's tie) can make that partner feel as special as they are to you. Nothing is more heartbreaking for many age players than seeing their Daddy calling someone else their little princess. If you choose to have multiple partners with whom you engage in roleplay, even if they all call you the same term, I highly recommend finding unique terms and pet names to call each of them. Someone in boy space could be a baby boy, little man, prince, precious… and so many other terms.

If you are playing with multiple adultz, I recommend this strategy as well. Unless you create a roleplay story where somehow you have three Mommies, it is hard for each Mommy to feel special. Many polyamorous or open relationships I know that engage in age play roles have a special role for each partner, and if the kidz want to have an age play scenario outside of their relationship core, ask that the Adultz take on non-threatening roles to the family dynamic, such as Doctor, Nurse, Teacher, or Uncle Phil.

Chapter Six. Negotiation and Organic Evolution.

There are many styles of negotiation out there. Some people enjoy taking a book like this one and highlighting what sounds hot to them, and handing it to their play partner. Others enjoy sitting face to face and talking about their desires. Perhaps talking online with a checklist is more your style? Maybe it's about curling up in bed after a hot night of fucking and whispering dirty fantasies in each other's ear? Either way, discussing and negotiating ahead of time is one of the easiest ways to avoid misunderstandings and heartache.

However, not every age play scene has an opportunity for formal negotiation. Perhaps, like me with my little boy, it started with a wink and a few words and the play began. Be aware that this kind of organic play style can be both rewarding and deeply frightening. What happened? Where do we go from here? Am I forcing my fantasy on my partner? All of these questions and more can come to mind, and I highly recommend sitting down some time after the scene with your play partner and checking in on what they thought of the scene. This kind of post-scene check-in offers the bottom a chance to speak up if anything didn't seem right, and the top a chance to be reassured if everything went well — both particularly important after an impromptu adventure.

Chapter Seven. Discipline and Punishment.

A common theme In a lot of age play porn is discipline and punishment. Discipline is usually not related directly to any specific behavior, and instead is any variety of tools to remind a person what their role is and how to behave. Punishment, on the other hand, is usually related directly to a specific activity, such as stealing a cookie or not doing homework, and it is pointed out that because you did this activity, you are getting this punishment. Not all discipline or punishment is physical, and can instead have a verbal, mental or social element. Verbal punishments can include yelling or polite talks about the fact that you knew better. Mental punishments can involve making you think about how that made your Daddy feel or writing assignments in your journal. Social punishments include not being allowed to play with specific people any more, or having to debase yourself in a semi-public setting, letting everyone know what you did wrong.

Discipline and punishment can be fun and hot, or can be deeply emotional and life-changing. I have known age players who use these tools to help their partners quit smoking, or modify other grown-up behaviors. Be careful doing this. Blurring the lines between age play and daily living is an advanced technique and should be done with care. In addition, I find that one major tool is left out that should be used more often in behavior modification — enforcement. Discipline or punishment after the fact is only so useful if no reinforcement or training was done ahead of time. Enforcement gives kidz cues as to whether or not their behavior is appropriate, and corrects it as soon as possible. "Good boy, that is exactly what I wanted," or "no, girl, do it this way," are great examples of verbal enforcement, but gold stars on a calendar when things were done right, or prizes as thanks for doing things right, are also great forms of physical enforcement.

Do you want to create a cowering individual who is always afraid of the cane or brush, or someone who wants to grow and become your prized partner? Punishment as fun roleplay can be very enjoyable, but take a minute and consider the ramifications of the play you are doing if it is part of a relationship where persona investment or 24-7 dynamics are involved.

Chapter Eight. Age Play Affects Outsiders.

Whether we like it or not, we do not live in a vacuum. What we do in our roleplay affects everyone who encounters it. Some may be inspired by the fun you are having and want to try it themselves. Others may be triggered by what they see you do as adults; they might have their own memories of childhood trauma and perceive that you are mocking them, hurting them, or mirroring the behavior of their own personal villains in your play life.

We can not change how others think or have gut reactions. We can, however, control our own behavior and how we react when this sort of reaction surfaces in someone else. Tactics I have used over the years include:

— Not doing overt age play in front of audiences who are likely to be offended (is doing that spanking the right thing to do at the grocery store?)

— Choosing backup pet names for public play (instead of Daddy, what about Papa Bear, their first or last name, or something else?)

— Politely pointing out that this is roleplay, not encouraging pedophilia or whatever else the confused spectator is likely offended by

— Showing people the sides of you outside of the age play scenario

— Offering to give questioners a copy of this book or other resources

— Understanding that people's baggage is their own, and we can only do so much, but we can be empathetic, sympathetic, and compassionate in our responses to their pain.

Chapter Nine. Not All Sunshine and Roses.

As we mentioned at the end of the last chapter, age play is not always sunshine and roses. The reality is that when we engage in age dynamic roleplay, we are opening up a huge potential can of worms — because unlike other sorts of erotic roleplay), every single one of us has actually been a child in the past. We all have baggage — some of us just have it packed differently than others. Whether you are hauling around three matching roller bags of emotional junk, or if you just have a handbag (with a handy storage locker in the back of your mind to keep the rest in, out of sight), we all have memories, so here are some key ideas to keep in mind as we open up this hot, fun, and sexy can of worms.

Therapeutic, not therapy

Age play can be incredibly therapeutic. Cathartic release of our past traumas, getting to dive into our fears and past memories while being supported by a loving partner, can help us reopen old wounds and examine them from the safety of the years between ourselves and our memories. However, age play is not therapy. There are accredited sex therapists who use rebirthing techniques, age roleplay and other similar concepts for helping individuals understand their past traumas and examine them in a therapy setting — but your partner is your partner, not your client. If, for example, you keep asking your lover to say a specific series of words while pinning you down and doing rape play with you, it might be worthwhile to examine whether this is still just hot fun roleplay, or whether this roleplay has touched on memories that would be better handled in a therapist's office.

The land mines

History is an amazing thing. We each carry around so much of it, and it affects every part of our life. How can we believe that it wouldn't affect our relationships, let alone our roleplay? "Land mines," also known as "triggers," are anything that may bring up bad memories, or are things we want to avoid in age play. For individuals with post-traumatic stress disorders, or other forms of trauma-related mental conditions, land mines are the things that pull the individual out of the fun roleplay and into a memory where their partner is no longer just their partner, but is now playing the role of a past perpetrator of trauma in their life.

Physical land mines can include specific types of touch, specific areas that feel wrong being touched during sexual play, objects that evoke bad memories, and specific wardrobe items for themselves or their partner that trigger unwanted reactions. If one of my partners asks me not to do a physical activity, I respect that request, and if it is something that I really want to do to fuel my own desires or fantasies, I will discuss it with them a few days later to find out what prompted the request they made.

Verbal land mines are also known as trigger words or trigger phrases. These verbal cues do not have to always be negative sounding ones like “shame on you,” as I have met some individuals whose childhood bullies used positive sounding words like “such a cute girl” every time they wanted to begin pushing them.

Not everyone knows they have land mines. Not everyone has land mines. In fact, I know people who have done age play for decades and never run into a land mine. I have also met individuals who on their first age play attempt ended up hitting their lover’s land mines with such force that their partner completely dissociated and was a broken mess. Thus, if you know you have land mines, please tell your play partner about them.. Discussion in advance, or polite requests to have your partner not do an activity if it starts or is brought up, can save everyone a lot of heartache. And if your partner makes requests, again, please respect them lest you be the one left to clean it all up afterwards.

Hot buttons and gifts from the past

Not all triggers are negative. Many of us carry around a lot of hot memories as well, and there are physical and verbal triggers that can plug us into our sexiness. For some people it is our partner slipping into a pair of seamed stockings or fishnets, because those were the first pieces of "naughty" lingerie we ever got to glimpse when we were children. For others it is a series of words our first lover whispered to us in bed, and when we hear them again the emotional sensations of early romance sweep back and we can go for the endorphin ride those words provide.

If you know some of your hot buttons, consider sharing them with your partner — or enjoy the fun you'll have finding them along the way!

If it all goes pear-shaped

I hope it will never happen to you, but sometimes, we humans break. I know I have in the past because of age play. Past memories have been triggered, and suddenly our partner is screaming, crying, or has gone completely silent in a dissociative fugue state. What do we do?

My first rule of thumb is to respect my partner's immediate desires as long as they are not put at physical risk by doing so. I know of individuals who have wanted to stop all roleplay on the spot and discuss exactly what happened. Even though breaking out of roleplay is a mood killer, hard-ons can be brought back; trust is much harder to rebuild. Others simply want to pause, have a minor behavior modified, and then keep going full speed ahead. Each person is different, and will ask for different things, if they can.

Unfortunately, if a full blown emotional land mine has been triggered, sometimes your partner may be a physical risk to themselves if left alone. Assess the situation. If they ask to be held, do so. If they ask to be left alone — is it safe to do so? If not, can you sit at the opposite side of the room and let them have some space? If they are in a catatonic state, perhaps you can just curl up and let them know that you are there — you, not whoever they may have slipped into believing you were for a moment.

Whether or not you ever have history of any sort surface, it is important to appreciate the power dynamics and unique vulnerabilities that this kind of play can create. Reccurring age play dynamics are powerfully intoxicating, and can become addictive for some individuals. Just try to remember that though we draw from childhood to inspire our fantasies, we are neither trying to recreate those memories or to create new childhood memories to replace previous ones.

Broken kidz/adultz — when others have come before

Not all our age play reactions come from childhood memories. If you have explored age play with other consenting adults, you have created memories as to what age play looks like. I have had some pretty powerful and amazing roleplay memories get smashed by hurtful real-world behavior on the part of my partner. This sort of problem can leave us feeling that we are not good enough boyz or girlz, not loving enough Daddies or Mommies, not desirable, not adequate.

If you have explored age play before and want to start doing so again with a new partner — remember that your new partner is not your old partner. They are a new relationship, so I suggst that you not treat them the exact same way you treated a previous one. Do not buy them the same toys, same wardrobe, or play out the exact same fantasies. Make this relationship as special as it deserves to be, and talk to them about where they want to go with this erotic roleplay. They deserve to be treated like the unique little snowflake that they are, so don't paint them with the same brush from your last relationship.

Also understand that objects hold power. If you were given an age-play-related prop by a previous relationship that has since ended, I highly recommend either having a ritual to claim it as your own, or giving it away. When someone gives us a gift, especially if we use that gift with them, we associate memories with that item and imbue that object with power related to that specific relationship dynamic. It is possible to cleanse that energy from an object, but it is hard work, so instead of tying to give your ex-girlfriend's wardrobe to your new girlfriend, consider giving those clothes away to someone you're not sexually involved with and go shopping with your new girlfriend — she'll likely feel far more special for getting to be part of the process with you!

Final Thoughts

Remember, each person has their own history, their own desires, and their own joys. Exploring those joys and desires with our lovers and play mates is incredibly powerful, and far more fulfilling than handing over a script to someone and asking them to read it back.

So what turns you on? What turns your partner on? How do you communicate your fantasies and desires to one another? Which of the ideas in this book really made you get all hot and bothered? Curious to give it a try once? Want to do over and over again?

Then curl up with your lover, write them a dirty note, throw on an apron or a pair of frog-print pajamas... and see where you can go together with the wide world of fantasy that is AGE PLAY.

Resources

Inspired? Want to take your exploration online to talk with other age players? Here is a list of a few websites I have enjoyed, but you can find more resources by exploring the internet.

Age and Role-Play Discussion
http://www.ageroleplay.idleplay.net/

Littles Group Documentation Project
http://www.theghidrah.com/lgdp/

Littles and Baby Pride Symbol
http://www.babypridestore.com/

Understanding Infantilism
http://understanding.infantilism.org/

Diaper Pail Fraternity
http://www.dpf.com/

Gloria's Age Play Link List
http://gloria-brame.com/kinkylinks/ageplay.html

Guardian Island Age Play Resort
http://www.ageplay.org/

Adult Baby Sitting Services
http://www.adultbabysitting.com/

LiveJournal Communities
http://www.livejournal.com
adultbabies, ageplay, ageplaydiscuss, ageplaywithsex, inner_nymphette, leather_girls, little_books, me_n_mommy, queer_daddy… and more!

BIOGRAPHY

Lee Harrington is an eclectic artist, spiritual and erotic educator, gender radical and published author on human sexuality and spiritual experience.

Part of the international sex positive communities since 1995, his stories make people laugh while showing you that eroticism can be as serious, sexy, or silly as you make it. Lee's writings and photography (also under a previous pen/porn name, Bridgett Harrington) have appeared in numerous publications, and his image has been seen everywhere from PlayboyTV to

SkinTwo. Learn more at www.PassionAndSoul.com.

OTHER BOOKS FROM

TOYBAG GUIDES: A Workshop In A Book *$9.95 each*

Canes and Caning, by Janet Hardy
Clips and Clamps, by Jack Rinella
Dungeon Emergencies & Supplies, by Jay Wiseman
Erotic Knifeplay, by Miranda Austin and Sam Atwood
Foot and Shoe Worship, by Midori
High-Tech Toys, by John Warren
Hot Wax and Temperature Play, by Spectrum
Medical Play, by Tempest

BDSM/KINK

The New Bottoming Book
The New Topping Book
both by Dossie Easton & Janet W. Hardy $14.95 ea.

The Compleat Spanker
Lady Green $12.95

Erotic Slavehood
Christina Abernathy $12.95

Erotic Tickling
Michael Moran $13.95

Family Jewels: A Guide to Male Genital Play and Torment
Hardy Haberman $12.95

Flogging
Joseph W. Bean $12.95

Intimate Invasions: The Ins and Outs of Erotic Enema Play
M.R. Strict $13.95

Jay Wiseman's Erotic Bondage Handbook
Jay Wiseman $16.95

The Kinky Girl's Guide to Dating
Luna Grey $16.95

The Loving Dominant
John Warren $16.95

The Mistress Manual: The Good Girl's Guide to Female Dominance
Mistress Lorelei $16.95

Please include $3 for first book and $1 for each additional book with your order to cover shipping and handling costs, plus $10 for overseas orders.
VISA/MC/Discover/AmEx accepted.

GREENERY PRESS

Play Piercing
Deborah Addington $13.95

Radical Ecstasy: SM Journeys to Transcendence
Dossie Easton and Janet W. Hardy $16.95

The Sexually Dominant Woman: A Workbook for Nervous Beginners
Lady Green $11.95

The Seductive Art of Japanese Bondage
Midori $27.95

SM 101: A Realistic Introduction
Jay Wiseman $24.95

GENERAL SEXUALITY

... But I Know What You Want: 25 Sex Tales for the Different
James Williams $13.95

The Ethical Slut: A Guide to Infinite Sexual Possibilities
Dossie Easton & Catherine A. Liszt $16.95

Fantasy Made Flesh: The Essential Guide to Erotic Roleplay
Deborah Addington $13.95

A Hand in the Bush: The Fine Art of Vaginal Fisting
Deborah Addington $13.95

Paying For It: A Guide By Sex Workers for Their Clients
edited by Greta Christina $13.95

Phone Sex: Oral Thrills and Aural Skills
Miranda Austin $15.95

Sex Disasters... And How to Survive Them
Charles Moser, Ph.D., M.D. and Janet W. Hardy $16.95

Tricks... To Please a Man
Tricks... To Please a Woman
both by Jay Wiseman $14.95 ea.

When Someone You Love Is Kinky
Dossie Easton & Catherine A. Liszt $15.95

CHECK OUR WEBSITE AT WWW.GREENERYPRESS.COM FOR HOT BDSM FICTION!

Order from Greenery Press, 4200 Park Blvd. pmb 240, Oakland, CA 94602, 510/530-1281. www.greenerypress.com.